Sameh Achoura
Cheddy Taamallah

CHRONIC ADULT HYDROCEPHALUS :

Sameh Achoura
Cheddy Taamallah

CHRONIC ADULT HYDROCEPHALUS :

PROGNOSTIC ELEMENTS OF SURGICAL MANAGEMENT

ScienciaScripts

Cover image: www.ingimage.com

This book is a translation from the original published under ISBN 978-620-6-72082-9.

Publisher:
Sciencia Scripts
is a trademark of
Dodo Books Indian Ocean Ltd. and OmniScriptum S.R.L publishing group

120 High Road, East Finchley, London, N2 9ED, United Kingdom
Str. Armeneasca 28/1, office 1, Chisinau MD-2012, Republic of Moldova, Europe
Printed at: see last page
ISBN: 978-620-8-05755-8

TABLE OF CONTENTS

INTRODUCTION

Previously known as normal pressure hydrocephalus (NPH), it has been known as chronic adult hydrocephalus (CAH) since the work of Bret and Chazal in the French-language literature in 1995 [1]. Chronic hydrocephalus in adults is a clinical syndrome classically characterised by gait disorders, dementia and urinary incontinence with radiological signs of ventricular dilatation without elevation of intracranial pressure (ICP) [2].

This clinical picture, which is often incomplete, usually presents late (up to the 6th or 7th decade). The pathophysiology of ventricular dilatation in CAH has yet to be explained. A change in cerebral compliance to the fluid pulse, an age-related disturbance in fluid resorption and vascular and genetic factors have been cited as possible causes [3]. In the presence of pathology of the central nervous system or trauma, chronic adult hydrocephalus is said to be secondary. In the absence of other causes, it is said to be primary or idiopathic [3].

The diagnosis of CAH is generally clinical. Alzheimer's disease remains the main differential diagnosis, which must be ruled out [4].

Magnetic resonance imaging (MRI) and cerebral computed tomography (CT) are used to confirm the diagnosis by showing ventricular dilatation and to rule out other pathologies of the central nervous system [5].

Given the variability of the clinical picture, the diagnosis of CAH remains a challenge for treating physicians, as does its management [6].Management is generally surgical, with the placement of a permanent fluid shunt resulting in a significant but sometimes temporary improvement in symptoms in most patients [7].However, there are few data in the literature concerning the prognostic factors for successful surgical management. The main aim of this study is therefore to determine the prognostic elements of the neurosurgical management of patients with chronic adult hydrocephalus.

METHODS

1. Design and framework of the study :

This was a retrospective, descriptive, monocentric study carried out in the neurosurgery department of the Hôpital Militaire Principal d'Instruction de Tunis (HMPIT) over a 16-year period (from 2004 to 2020).

2. Study population :

2.1. Inclusion criteria :

Our study included all patients over 40 years of age who were admitted to the neurosurgery department of the Hôpital Militaire Principal d'Instruction de Tunisie from 2004 to 2020 for treatment of chronic adult hydrocephalus.

Non-inclusion criteria :

All subjects with malformations of a different location in the brain or with hydrocephalus with intracranial hypertension were not included.

Exclusion criteria :

Patients under 40 years of age were excluded from the study, and four patients initially included were excluded for lack of data.

3. Primary endpoint:

This study focuses on the occurrence of at least one episode of recurrence in order to determine the risk factors for recurrence in patients operated on for chronic adult hydrocephalus.

4. Data collection :

The following information was collected on an electronic database for each patient admitted to the neurosurgery department of the Hôpital Militaire Principal d'Instruction de Tunis between 2004 and 2020:

Basic features

Age and gender.

Medical history: neurosurgical, neurological, diabetes, cardiovascular disease.

Diagnostic tests of HPN

Imaging: Cerebral CT scan and cerebral MRI. Depletive lumbar puncture.

Symptomatology

The symptoms presented by the patient at the time of admission and their evolution over time: gait and balance problems, urinary incontinence, dementia syndrome, visual disturbance, headaches and altered state of consciousness.

Evolution

Improvement and post-operative complications, recurrences and subsequent evolution in the 02 years post-operatively were collected.

5. Analysis statistics

We used IBM SPSS version 23 to create the database and the tables. Microsoft Excel was used to produce the graphs. The results of the qualitative and quantitative variables were expressed respectively as a mean and as a percentage (or headcount (n)). The significance level was set at p ::; 0.05.

6. Ethical considerations and conflict of interest

Given the retrospective nature of the analysis, written informed consent was waived. The data collected from patients was rendered anonymous after analysis. Only the file identification number was recorded for possible verification. No conflicts of interest were declared for this study.

7. Bibliographic Research :

The search engines used for bibliographic research were: Pubmed and Google Scholar. The keywords used were: Normal pressure hydrocephalus-Outcome-Prognosis. ZOTERO software was used to enter and organise the references.

RESULTS

A. Descriptive study

I. EPIDEMIOLOGICAL CHARACTERISTICS

Between 2004 and 2020, 52 patients were admitted to the neurosurgery department of the Hôpital Militaire Principal d'Instruction de Tunis, of whom 06 were excluded. Of the 46 patients initially included, 40 were retained. Figure 1 shows the diagram of the study.

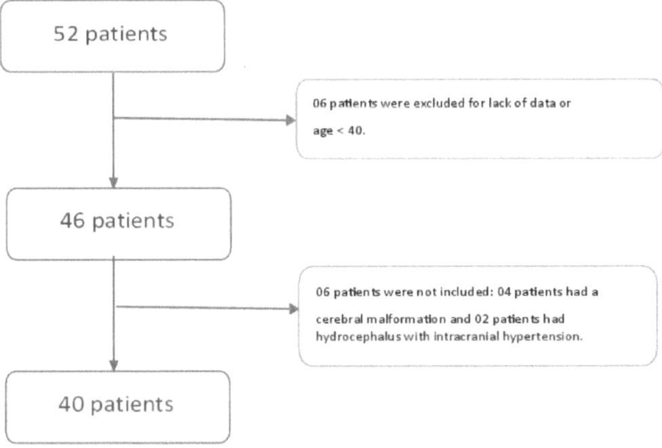

Figure 1: Diagram of the study

1. Frequency :

The annual frequency of patients presenting with chronic adult hydrocephalus is 2.5 patients per year with an increase in the number of patients since the year 2018 with a peak of 06 patients : Figure 2.

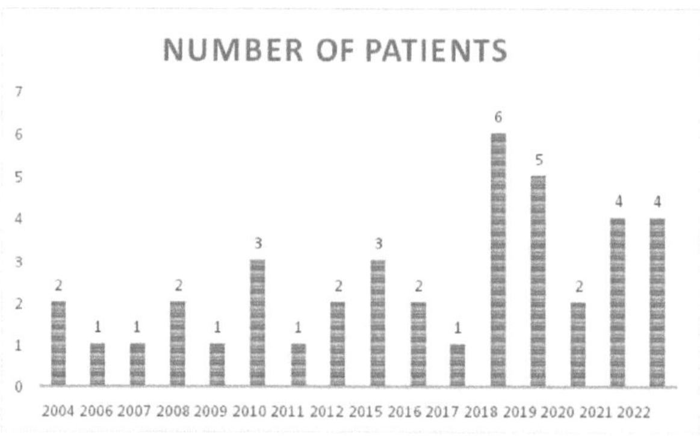

Figure 2: Patient frequency by year

2. Age:

The average age of the patients was 69, ranging from 44 to 83.

The average age for men was 69. For women, it was 73.

The 74 to 83 age group was the most affected, with 18 patients (45%): Table I.

Table I: Patient frequency by year.

Age range	44 - 63	64- 73	74 - 83
Number of cases	10	12	18
Percentage	25 %	30 %	45 %

3. Sex :

There were 17 female patients (42.5%) and 23 male patients (57.5%). The sex ratio was 1.35: Figure 3.

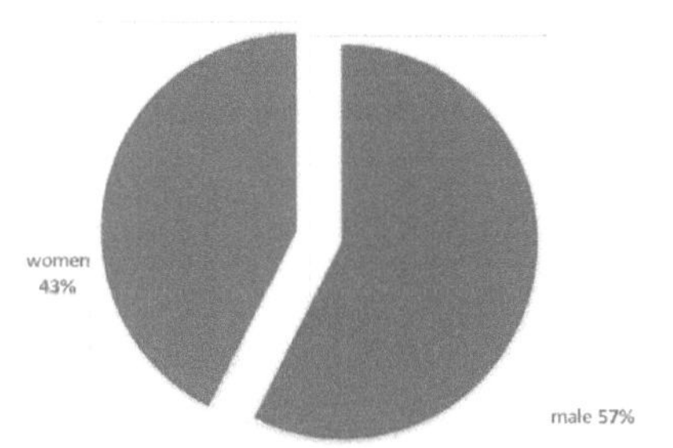

Figure 3: Breakdown of patients by gender

II.CHARACTERISTICS CLINICAL

1. Development time

The duration of evolution is the time between the appearance of the first clinical signs and the patient's consultation leading to hospitalisation and treatment.

The average duration of the disease was 15 months, with extremes ranging from 01 months to 05 years.

2. Revealing mode

The onset of the disease was monosymptomatic in 07 patients, i.e. 17.5% of cases, 11 patients had 02 elements of the CAII triad, i.e. 27.5% of cases, and 22 patients had the complete triad, i.e. 55% of cases.

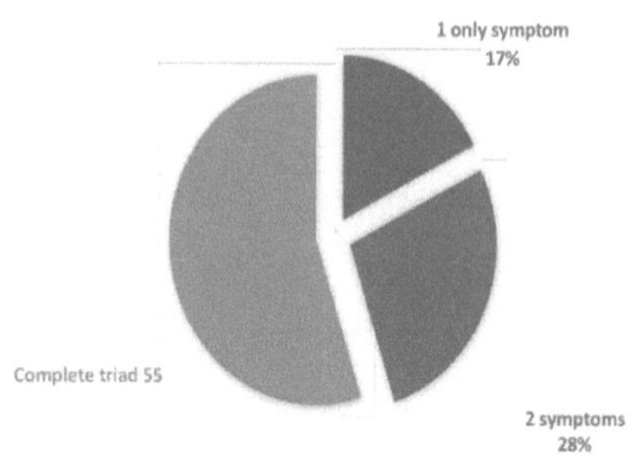

Figure 4: How the disease is revealed

3. Clinical signs (Table 2)

3.1. Adams and Hakim triad

- Gait disorders accounted for 92.5% of cases (37 cases).

- Urinary incontinence accounted for 67.5% of cases (27 cases).

- The dementia syndrome was present in 77.5% of cases, i.e. 31 cases.

- The Adams and Hakim triad was complete in 22 patients in our series, i.e. 55% of cases.

11 patients presented 2 signs of the triad: 06 patients presented gait disorders and a dementia syndrome, i.e. 15% of cases, 04 patients presented gait disorders and urinary incontinence, i.e. 10% of cases, and only 1 patient presented urinary incontinence and a dementia syndrome, i.e. 2.5% of cases. 09 patients presented only 1 sign of the triad: 05 patients presented only gait disorders, i.e. 12.5% of cases, 02 patients presented an isolated dementia syndrome, i.e. 5% of cases, and no patient presented isolated urinary incontinence. Figure 5.

3.2. Other clinical signs

In the study, patients presented with clinical signs other than the Adams and Hakim triad:

- 10 patients had headaches, i.e. 25% of cases.
- 7 patients (17.5%) had visual problems.
- 6 patients suffered from vertigo (15% of cases).
- 5 patients presented with behavioural problems, i.e. 12.5% of cases.
- 1 patient had a convulsive seizure (2.5% of cases)

Table II: Clinical signs in our series

Clinical signs	Number of cases	Percentage
Walking disorders	37	92.5%
Dementia syndrome	31	77.5%
Urinary incontinence	27	67.5%
Headaches	10	25%
Visual disorders	07	17.5%
Dizziness	06	15%
Behavioural problems	05	12.5%
Convulsive seizures	01	2.5%

4. Pathological history

- 05 patients had a history of stroke (12.5% of cases).
- 02 patients had a history of Parkinson's disease (5% of cases).
- 03 patients had a history of CAH (7.5% of cases).

• 01 patient had a history of meningeal haemorrhage (2.5% of cases).

• 02 patients (5%) had a history of chronic subdural haematoma.

• 22 patients had arterial hypertension (55% of cases).

• 15 patients (37.5%) had type 2 diabetes.

• 07 patients had dyslipidaemia, i.e. 17.5% of cases.

• 05 patients with coronary artery disease stenosis were treated with Aspegic (12.5% of cases).

• 04 patients had chronic renal failure, i.e. 10% of cases.

In addition, 4 patients had no previous pathological history, i.e. 10% of cases.

Table III: Breakdown of patients by history.

MEDICAL HISTORY	Number of cases	Percentage
AVC	05	12.5%
Parkinson's disease	02	5%
HCA	03	7.5%
Meningeal haemorrhage	01	2.5%
Chronic HSD	02	5%
HTA	22	55%
Type 2 diabetes	15	37.5%
Dyslipidemia	07	17.5%
Stenotic coronary artery disease	05	12.5%
IRC	04	10%

III. PARACLINICAL EXAMINATIONS

1. Brain imaging

Brain imaging was performed in all patients in the series. They received either brain computed tomography (cTc) or brain magnetic resonance imaging (cMRI). The diagnosis was confirmed by imaging in all patients.

Cerebral CT

CT scans were performed on 20 patients, i.e. 50% of cases.

12 patients had triventricular dilatation, i.e. 60%, while 08 patients had quadriventricular dilatation, i.e. 40%.

Brain MRI

28 patients underwent cMRI, i.e. 70% of cases. (06 patients also benefited from a CT scan).

19 patients had triventricular dilatation (68%) and 09 patients had quadriventricular dilatation (32%).

A total of 28 patients had triventricular dilatation on either cT or cMRI, i.e. 70% of the cases in the study, compared with 12 patients with quadriventricular dilatation, i.e. 30% of the cases in the study (Figure 5).

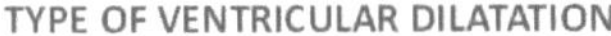

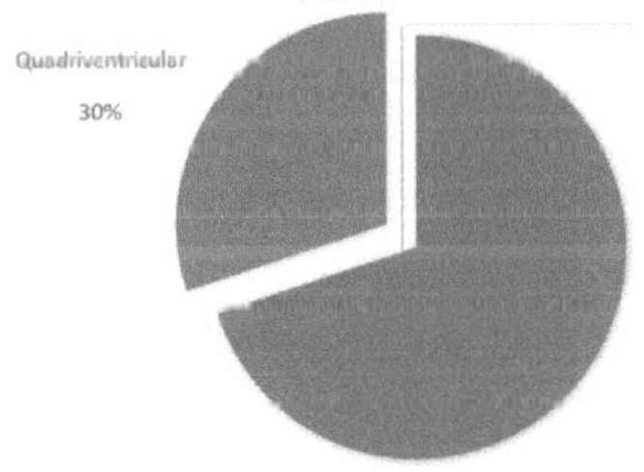

Figure 5: Type of ventricular dilation

Lumbar puncture

Lumbar puncture (LP) was performed in 26 patients (65% of cases).

13 patients received a single LP, i.e. 50% of cases. 05 patients underwent 2 lumbar punctures, i.e. 19% of cases.

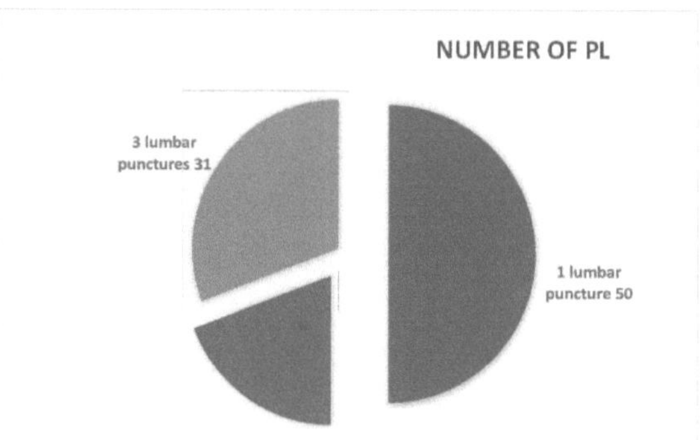

Figure 6: Number of LPs performed for each patient 08 patients underwent 3 lumbar punctures, i.e. 31% of cases. (Figure 6).

IV. TREATMENT

39 patients in the study underwent surgical treatment (97.5%). Only one patient did not undergo surgery due to the non-negligible risk of surgery (2.5%). 37 patients were treated with a ventriculoperitoneal shunt (VPS), i.e. 95% of cases, and 2 patients were treated with a ventriculocisternostomy (VCS), i.e. 5% of cases.

V. EVOLUTION

1. Intraoperative incidents

All patients underwent surgery without any intraoperative incidents.

2. Post-operative course

2.1. Post-operative complications

5 patients had postoperative complications, i.e. 13% of cases.

• 1 patient had bacterial meningitis which was treated with antibiotics and improved immediately.

• 1 patient presented with a generalised tonic-clonic epileptic seizure and was put on anti-epileptic treatment without any recurrence of seizures.

• 1 patient had an extra-peritoneal catheter requiring re-insertion.

• 2 patients had valve dysfunction requiring valve replacement.

Table IV: Types of post-operative complications

Type of complications	Number of cases
Bacterial meningitis	01
Epileptic seizure	01
Extra-peritoneal catheter	01
Valve malfunction	02

2.2. Immediate development

• Gait disorders: Of the 33 patients with gait disorders, 32 underwent surgery, including 2 with VCS. The immediate outcome was favourable in 71% of patients, with disappearance of gait disorders.

• Urinary incontinence: Of the 27 patients with urinary incontinence, 26 underwent surgery, including 1 patient with VCS. The immediate outcome was favourable in 47% of patients with disappearance of urinary incontinence.

• Dementia: All patients with dementia underwent DVP surgery. The immediate outcome was favourable in 44% of patients, with disappearance of the dementia syndrome.

3. Recurrences

Of the 39 patients who underwent surgery, 12 (30%) had a recurrence of CAH.

- 2 patients recurred between 01 and 03 months, i.e. 17% of cases.
- 1 patient recurred between 03 and 06 months, i.e. 08% of cases.
- 1 patient recurred between 06 and 12 months, i.e. 08% of cases.
- 5 patients relapsed between 12 and 24 months, i.e. 42% of cases.
- 3 patients had a recurrence lasting > 24 months, i.e. 25% of cases.

Gait disorders: Gait disorders reappeared in 8 patients, i.e. 67% of cases.

Urinary incontinence: Urinary incontinence reappeared in 3 patients, i.e. 25% of cases.

Dementia syndrome: Dementia syndrome reappeared in 4 patients (33% of cases).

Table V: Number of patients with recurrence and time to recurrence

Time limit for repeat offences	Number of patients	Percentage
01-03 months	02	17%
03-06 months	01	08%
06-12 months	01	08%
12-24 months	05	42%
>24 months	03	25%

4. Resume surgery

Of the 39 patients operated on, 7 (18%) required repeat surgery.

• 1 patient had an extra-peritoneal catheter requiring re-insertion.

• 2 patients had valve malfunction requiring valve replacement.

• 4 patients had a recurrence of clinical signs of CAH requiring revision

5. Deaths

Of the patients initially included in the study, 7 (17.5%) died. Only 1 patient died in the department following cardiorespiratory arrest after 2 weeks. 2 patients died between 12 and 24 months later. 1 patient died following an infectious pneumopathy with no improvement in the clinical signs of CAH. The other patient died following a COVID-19 infection with a clear improvement in the clinical signs of CAH. 4 patients died within >24 months. 2 patients died of ischaemic stroke. 1 patient died following a COVID-19 infection and the other patient died following a stroke. All of these patients showed partial improvement in clinical signs: 3 patients retained a slight walking disorder and 1 patient retained urinary incontinence.

B. Analytical study

The study population was divided into two groups:

- Patients who had an optimal outcome

- Patients who had a non-optimal outcome

Following a test of the clinical and radiological variables, we compared the statistical relationship between the optimal evolution of patients two years after surgical treatment and the pre-established variables.

I. Univariate study

1. Age and sex

In our study, we found that there was no statistically significant relationship between optimal outcome and patient age (**p=0.964**).

There was no statistically significant relationship between optimal outcome and patient gender (**p=0.969**).

2. History

In our study, we found that 66.6% of patients who had a recurrence were hypertensive and 50% of patients who had an optimal outcome were hypertensive. However, there was no statistically significant relationship between hypertension and optimal outcome (**p=0.350**).

There was no statistically significant relationship between diabetes and optimal outcome (**p=0.768**). Thus, 33.3% of patients who relapsed were diabetic and 39.3% of patients with optimal outcome were diabetic.There was no statistically significant relationship between other comorbidities and optimal outcome.

3. Development time

We found that there was a statistically significant relationship between duration of progression and optimal progression (**p=0.03**). Thus, 58.3% of patients who relapsed had a disease course of more than 24 months. In fact, the time between the appearance of the first clinical signs and surgical management was 8 months for patients who had an optimal course, compared with 25 months for patients who relapsed.

4. Type of dilatation ventricular

We found that there was no statistically significant relationship between the type of ventricular dilatation, either tri-ventricular or quadri-ventricular, and optimal outcome (**p=0.523**).

5. Number of punctures lumbar

In our study, we found that there was a statistically significant relationship between the number of lumbar punctures and optimal outcome (**p=0.029**). Thus, 100% of patients who had 3 lumbar punctures did not relapse, compared with 83% of patients with a non-optimal course who had only one lumbar puncture or none at all, as shown in Table 4.

Table VI: Statistical relationships between the number of HGVs and optimal development

Optimum patient outcomes

No (n=12)			Yes (n=28)	
Number of HGVs	n	%	n	%
0	5	41.6%	9	32%
1	5	41.6%	8	28.6%
2	2	16.6%	3	10.7%
3	0	0%	8	28.6%

6. Treatment surgical

In our study, we did not find a statistically significant relationship between optimal patient outcome and the type of bypass.

7. Post-operative complications

We found that in our study, there was a statistically significant relationship between the absence of post operative complications and optimal patient outcome (**p=0.024**). Indeed, of the 5 patients who had post-operative complications, 4 (80%) had recurrences.

DISCUSSION

I. Main results of our study

This is a retrospective study of 40 patients treated for CAH over a 16-year period (from 2004 to 2020).

At the time of diagnosis, the average age of patients was 69, ranging from 44 to 83. The 74 to 83 age group was the most affected, with a frequency of 45%. The sex ratio was 1.35. 90% of our population had at least one comorbidity.

Hypertension and diabetes were the most common medical conditions (55% and 37.5% respectively).

The average duration of the disease was 15 months. 55% of our population had the complete Adams and Hakim triad.

The most frequent symptom was gait disturbance, with a frequency of 92.5%.

All patients underwent brain imaging.

Brain MRI was the most commonly used imaging modality in 70% of our population. Tri-ventricular dilatation was determined in 70% of our population and quadri-ventricular dilatation in 30% of our population.

At least one lumbar puncture was performed in 65% of our population.

Surgical treatment was performed in 97.5% of our population, except in one patient because of the non-negligible risk of surgery.

13% of patients who underwent surgery suffered post-operative complications.

The immediate evolution of gait disorders was favourable in all patients, with disappearance of the disorders. For urinary incontinence, the immediate outcome was favourable in 80% of patients. For the dementia syndrome, the immediate outcome was favourable in 47% of patients.

Of the patients who underwent surgery, 30% recurred. Gait disturbance was the most frequent symptom.18% of patients who underwent surgery required a second operation. Of the patients initially included in the study, 7 (17.5%) died. The univariate study showed that :

- The duration of disease progression had a statistically significant relationship with optimal progression (**p=0.03**).
- The number of depletive lumbar punctures had a statistically significant relationship with optimal outcome (**p=0.029**).
- The absence of complications in the immediate post-operative period had a statistically significant relationship with optimal outcome (**p=0.024**).

II. Strengths and limitations of our work

Our study has several strong points:

- According to our research, this is the first thesis on this subject anational level, and studies on the subject in Tunisia are rare.
- All the clinical and radiological characteristics of this condition were established in the descriptive study. The analytical study identified the prognostic elements of the neurosurgical management of chronic adult hydrocephalus.
- This work is one of the few studies to examine the factors that may cause recurrence of this condition.

However, our study has certain limitations:

- Some patients were lost to follow-up after discharge.
- Given the retrospective nature of the study, optimal data collection was not possible.

• The mono-centric nature of our work does not allow us to study a wider population.

III. Epidemiological data

1. Frequency :

Several hospital studies carried out in Germany [8], Norway [9] and the United States [10] have reported an incidence of CAH of 0.84 to 1.8 patients per 100,000 inhabitants per year. In our study, the annual incidence of patients with CAH was 2.5 per year. A Norwegian outpatient study of a population of 220,000 showed an incidence of 5.5 per 100,000 inhabitants per year.[11]. This shows that CAH is a condition that may be under-diagnosed [12].

2. Age :

In our study, the average age of the patients was 69, ranging from 44 to 83 years. The average age of women was 73 and of men 69. Our results are in line with the study by F Hertel et al [13] with a mean age of 69.2 years, ranging from 39 to 82 years.

3. Sex :

In our study, 57.5% of patients were male, with a sex ratio of 1.35. There is a slight difference between the percentage of women and men in the literature. In the studies carried out by F Hertel et al [13] and Klassen et al [10], there is a predominance of men. However, in the studies by Woodworth et al [14] and Algin et al [15], women predominate.

IV. CLINICAL DATA :

1. Development time

The time taken for the disease to progress is the time between the appearance of the first clinical signs and the patient's consultation leading to hospitalisation and treatment. In our study, the average duration of evolution in our patients was 15 months, with extremes ranging from 01 months to 5 years. We found that in several studies of CAH, the average duration of evolution was between 22 and 28 months [16] [17] [18].

2. Revealing mode

The clinical picture of chronic hydrocephalus in adults is characterised by an insidious and progressive onset and is clinically revealed by the ADAMS and HAKIM clinical triad combining gait disorders, urinary incontinence and dementia syndrome [19].

The onset of the disease may be monosymptomatic, bi-symptomatic or even a complete triad. The modes of onset differ from one study to another in the literature. In several studies, the complete triad is often present at the time of diagnosis. In the article by R. Nassar et al [20], 60% of patients presented with this triad. In our study, 55% of patients had the complete triad.

3. Clinical signs

Walking disorders

In patients with CAH, walking difficulties are the earliest and most frequent symptom [21] [22].

They are characterised by postural instability, difficulty in initiating walking or walking with small steps [23]. Our study showed that gait disorders were present in 92.5% of cases.

Incontinence

Unlike walking disorders and cognitive impairment, there is no clear recommendation as to the characteristics of urinary disorders [7]. In a study by Savolainen et al [23], the frequency of urinary incontinence was 49%. Another study by Krzastek et al [24] showed a frequency of 74.5% of cases with urinary incontinence.Our study showed that urinary incontinence was present in 67.5% of cases.

Dementia syndrome

Patients generally present with a depressive syndrome, psychomotor retardation and concentration and memory problems [25]. In our study, 77.5% of patients presented with a dementia syndrome, which is in line with the study by Bech et al [26] showing that dementia was present in 77% of cases.

4. Pathological history

In our study, the most common pathological histories in our patients were arterial hypertension and diabetes.22 patients in our series, i.e. 55%, had arterial hypertension. This is consistent with studies by Kobayashi et al [27] and Pyykkö et al [28] showing that 57% and 52% of patients respectively were hypertensive. The incidence of diabetes was 37.5% in our study. The study by Jacobs L [29] shows that 51.5% of patients included in the study were diabetic. This study is similar to that of Mirzayan et al [30], with a frequency of 51%. Other studies such as Israelsson et al [31] and Pyykkö et al [28] showed a lower frequency of 26.8% and 23% respectively.

V. PARACLINICAL EXAMINATIONS

1. Imaging

According to Japanese recommendations [7], the diagnosis of chronic adult hydrocephalus is based on clinical signs and ventricular dilatation on cerebral MRI or cerebral CT with an EVANS Index >0.3. In our study, all patients underwent brain imaging. 50% of patients had a brain scan and 70% had a brain MRI.We have noted that there have been no studies comparing the efficacy of cerebral CT versus cerebral MRI for the diagnosis of CAH. However, brain MRI remains the reference examination because it can reveal other associated pathologies and eliminate differential diagnoses [32].

Given the retrospective nature of our study, we have no detailed data on other lesions or imaging abnormalities. 70% of patients in our study had triventricular dilatation on imaging and 30% had quadriventricular dilatation.

2. Lumbar puncture

Lumbar puncture is a therapeutic test frequently used to confirm the diagnosis of CAH [7] and to identify patients who may have a favourable outcome after surgical treatment [33] . 65% of patients in our study had at least one lumbar puncture. 50% of these patients received a single LP, 19% received 2 LPs and 31% received 3 LPs.In a study by Lim et al [34], repeated lumbar punctures were suggested as an alternative treatment for patients who could not be operated on with ventricular bypass, with favourable improvement for at least one year after the last lumbar puncture.

VI. TREATMENT

There are several treatment options for chronic hydrocephalus in adults. Refraining from treatment, lumbar puncture for evacuation, medical treatment and surgical treatment can all be considered, depending on the severity of the symptoms and the patient's general condition. Surgical treatment by CSF shunting remains the gold standard and the most effective treatment [7] [25] [35].Ventriculoperitoneal shunting is the most frequently used shunt in the surgical treatment of CAH [36] [37]. 97.5% of patients in our study underwent surgical treatment. Only one patient did not undergo surgery due to the lack of benefit and the non-negligible risk of surgery.95% of patients operated on received a ventriculoperitoneal shunt (PVS) and 5% of patients operated on received a ventriculocisternostomy (VCS). Our results are in agreement with the study by Komolafe et al [37] which showed that 95.4% of patients were operated on by DVP and 4.6% by VCS. All our patients were fitted with a programmable valve, in line with the latest Japanese recommendations [7].

VII. POST-OPERATIVE EVOLUTION

1. Immediate post-operative

Several studies have discussed the immediate post-operative course using several methods to assess patients after surgical treatment, based mainly on clinical improvement [38].

In our study, the evaluation was based on the subjective clinical improvement of symptoms: gait disorders, urinary incontinence and dementia syndrome.

To the best of our knowledge, there are few studies on the immediate post-operative evolution of clinical symptoms. In terms of outcome, 87% of patients had a favourable outcome, either partial or total. 42% of patients operated on had a clear improvement in clinical signs in the immediate post-operative period and 45% of patients operated on had a partial improvement in clinical signs.

In our study, the immediate outcome was favourable in 71% of patients with walking difficulties, in 47% of patients with urinary incontinence and in 44% of patients with dementia.

2. Post-operative complications

The frequency of post-operative complications varies from study to study. The most frequent complications are central nervous system infections, cerebral haematomas, epileptic seizures and shunt obstruction [39] [40]. In our study, 13% of patients who underwent surgery suffered post-operative complications.

3. Recurrences

Improvement after bypass is generally limited in time. Several studies have shown that there is an overall deterioration after between 36 and 60 months [41].

In our study, we defined recurrence as a recurrence or worsening of clinical signs within a period of 2 years. 30% of our patients had a recurrence, with a predominance between 12 and 24 months. These results are similar to those of Tissel et al. al [42], showing that 21% of patients showed a worsening of clinical signs compared with signs before bypass.

4. Resume surgery

Of the 12 patients who had a recurrence, 07 underwent revision surgery, representing 18% of cases in our study. These results are similar to those of the study by Hebb et al [43], with 22% of patients requiring repeat surgery or revision of the shunt.

5. Deaths

CAH was not the cause of any deaths among the patients in our study. 17.5% of the patients initially included in the study died as a result of various pathologies: infectious pneumonitis, COVID-19, ischaemic stroke, stroke.

VIII. Analytical study

The study of prognostic factors for an optimal post-operative course of CAH has been carried out using various methods in different articles in the literature and not on the same standardisation bases [44] [45] [46].

According to our study, there is a statistically significant association between length of evolution and postoperative evolution (p=0.03). Our study concurs with those of Kimura et al (p=0.0015) [47] and Vakili et al (p=0.033) [18] who reported that a long duration of symptom progression is associated with deterioration after 06 or 1 year according to the mRS scale. Depletive lumbar puncture has been considered in several studies to be a criterion for the diagnosis of CAH and a prognostic factor for the success of shunting in patients with CAH. Improvement in clinical signs after LP is a good prognostic factor for post-operative outcome [48] [49] [50]. However, depletive LP has a lower sensitivity and specificity than continuous drainage [14] [51]. Continuous drainage is used less frequently, given its invasive and technical nature [52].

In our study, there was a statistically significant relationship between the number of depletive lumbar punctures and optimal outcome (p=0.029). In fact, none of the patients who received 03 LPs relapsed. Our results are in line with the study by Ishikawa et al [53] which suggests that repetitive lumbar punctures may have similar physiological effects to continuous drainage. Another study by da Rocha et al [54] shows that repetitive lumbar punctures increase the sensitivity of depletive lumbar puncture and bring it closer to the sensitivity of continuous drainage. With regard to the relationship between the occurrence of complications in the immediate post-operative period and the occurrence of recurrences, our study showed that there was a statistically significant relationship (p=0.024). To the best of our knowledge, there are currently no studies that have investigated the relationship between the occurrence of complications and subsequent recurrences. This lack of data may be explained by the fact that the pathophysiology of CAH is not well detailed [54]. With regard to cardiovascular pathologies, our study did not show a statistically significant relationship between the presence of vascular comorbidities and optimal outcome. This is in line with the results of studies by Andrén et al [55]. and Klinge et al [56] showing that the presence of cardiovascular risk factors is not correlated with optimal outcome.

CONCLUSIONS

Chronic adult hydrocephalus is a rare condition that mainly affects elderly subjects. Diagnosis is primarily clinical. It is characterised by the Adams and Hakim triad (gait disorders, urinary incontinence and dementia), but sometimes the clinical picture is incomplete.Given the variability of the clinical picture and the absence of an international consensus on the criteria for objective assessment of clinical signs, diagnosis remains a challenge for doctors, particularly front-line doctors.Imaging is a means of diagnostic certainty and a means of eliminating other differential diagnoses, as well as differentiating between idiopathic and secondary CAH. Depletive lumbar puncture is a therapeutic test for confirming the positive diagnosis of CAH and a prognostic factor for good outcome after surgical treatment.Treatment by ventricular bypass remains the gold standard. Ventriculoperitoneal shunting is the most commonly used type of shunt.However, few studies have looked at the prognostic factors for successful surgical management. Our study is a retrospective, descriptive and monocentric study carried out in the neurosurgery department of the Hôpital Militaire Principal d'Instruction de Tunis (HMPIT) over a period of 16 years (from 2004 to 2020). The primary endpoint of our study was the occurrence of at least one episode of recurrence up to 2 years after surgery.We included 40 patients, 39 of whom underwent surgery. The mean age on admission was 69 years. The 74 to 83 age group was the most affected, with a frequency of 45%. A predominance of men was noted, with a sex ratio of 1.35. 90% of our population had at least one comorbidity. The most frequent pathological antecedents were arterial hypertension and diabetes, with a frequency of 55% and 37.5% respectively. On admission, 55% of patients presented with the complete Adams and Hakim triad. Gait disturbance was the most frequent symptom with a frequency of 92.5%. Duration of evolution The mean duration of clinical signs was 15 months. All patients underwent brain imaging and the majority of patients showed triventricular dilatation with a frequency of 70%. At least one lumbar puncture as a therapeutic test was performed in 65% of patients.All but one of the patients underwent surgery because of the significant risk involved. Post-operative complications occurred in 13% of patients. The immediate outcome was favourable in the majority of patients. However, 30% of patients who underwent surgery had a recurrence. Walking difficulties were the most frequent symptom. 18% of operated patients required repeat surgery. As for mortality, none of the patients died as a result of CAH. The duration of disease progression (p=0.03), the number of depletive lumbar punctures (p=0.029) and the occurrence of post-operative complications (p=0.024) were good prognostic factors for the optimal outcome after shunting.Numerous studies have been carried out to assess the pathophysiological, clinical and radiological characteristics of chronic adult hydrocephalus, as well as the prognostic factors relating to the optimal course after surgical management. The lack of a standard GOLD for assessing clinical signs and the diversity of patient follow-up methods make it more difficult to study prognostic factors. In the course of this work :

- We emphasise the importance of using objective assessment scales for clinical signs before and after surgical treatment in order to be able to compare patients' progress objectively.

- In view of the lack of Tunisian studies on chronic adult hydrocephalus, we propose to carry out a multicentre study involving all Tunisian neurology and neurosurgery departments, in order to specify the epidemiological, clinical and radiological characteristics and to study the risk factors and prognostic factors in Tunisian patients.

- We insist on informing doctors on 1ère line and doctors the importance of diagnosing chronic adult hydrocephalus in order to prevent the disease from progressing over a long period.

On the basis of these results, we propose the following course of action:

- Assessment of the symptoms of chronic adult hydrocephalus using the scales proposed in the Japanese Guidelines in order to have objective assessment scales that are common to all services in Tunisia so as to be able to assess the evolution of patients after surgical management (appendices 1 and 2).

- Several lumbar punctures to optimise post-operative progress

- Educating patients and their families to increase their knowledge of chronic adult hydrocephalus and the importance of consulting a doctor as soon as clinical signs appear, so as to avoid trivialising the symptoms reported by the patient.

REFERENCES

1. P B, J C. Chronic ("normal pressure") hydrocephalus in childhood and adolescence. A review of 16 cases and reappraisal of the syndrome. Childs Nerv Syst ChNS Off J Int Soc Pediatr Neurosurg [Internet]. 1995 Dec [cited 2024 Feb 1];11(12). Available from: https://pubmed.ncbi.nlm.nih.gov/8750950/

2. Gavrilov GV, Gaydar BV, Svistov DV, Korovin AE, Samarcev IN, Churilov LP, Tovpeko DV. Idiopathic Normal Pressure Hydrocephalus (Hakim-Adams Syndrome): Clinical Symptoms, Diagnosis and Treatment. Psychiatr Danub. Dec 2019;31(Suppl 5):737-44.

3. Skalický P, Mládek A, Vlasák A, De Lacy P, Beneš V, Bradác O. Normal pressure hydrocephalus-an overview of pathophysiological mechanisms and diagnostic procedures. Neurosurg Rev. Dec 2020;43(6):1451-64.

4. Greenberg ABW, Mekbib KY, Mehta NH, Kiziltug E, Duy PQ, Smith HR, Junkkari A, Leinonen V, Hyman BT, Chan D, Curry WT, Arnold SE, Barker Ii FG, Frosch MP, Kahle KT. Utility of cortical tissue analysis in normal pressure hydrocephalus. Cereb Cortex N Y N 1991. 24 Jan 2024;bhae001.

5. Williams MA, Malm J. Diagnosis and Treatment of Idiopathic Normal Pressure Hydrocephalus. Contin Lifelong Learn Neurol. Apr 2016;22(2 Dementia):579-99.

6. Oliveira LM, Nitrini R, Román GC. Normal-pressure hydrocephalus. A critical review. Dement Neuropsychol. 2019;13(2):133-43.

7. NAKAJIMA M, YAMADA S, MIYAJIMA M, ISHII K, KURIYAMA N, KAZUI H, KANEMOTO H, SUEHIRO T, YOSHIYAMA K, KAMEDA M, KAJIMOTO Y, MASE M, MURAI H, KITA D, KIMURA T, SAMEJIMA N, TOKUDA T, KAIJIMA M, AKIBA C, KAWAMURA K, ATSUCHI M,

HIRATA Y, MATSUMAE M, SASAKI M, YAMASHITA F, AOKI S, IRIE R, MIYAKE H, KATO T, MORI E, ISHIKAWA M, DATE I, ARAI H. Guidelines for Management of Idiopathic Normal Pressure Hydrocephalus (Third Edition): Endorsed by the Japanese Society of Normal Pressure Hydrocephalus. Neurol Med Chir (Tokyo). Feb 2021;61(2):63-97.

8. Krauss JK, Halve B. Normal pressure hydrocephalus: survey on contemporary diagnostic algorithms and therapeutic decision-making in clinical practice. Acta Neurochir (Wien). Apr 2004;146(4):379-88; discussion 388.

9. A B, Hl F, S S, T M, T S, Pk E. Five-year incidence of surgery for idiopathic normal pressure hydrocephalus in Norway. Acta Neurol Scand [Internet]. Nov 2009 [cited 14 Sept 2023];120(5). Available at: https://pubmed.ncbi.nlm.nih.gov/19832773/

10. Klassen BT, Ahlskog JE. Normal pressure hydrocephalus: how often does the diagnosis hold water? Neurology. 20 Sep 2011;77(12):1119-25.

11. Brean A, Eide PK. Prevalence of probable idiopathic normal pressure hydrocephalus in a Norwegian population. Acta Neurol Scand. July 2008;118(1):48-53.

12. Martín-Láez R, Caballero-Arzapalo H, López-Menéndez LÁ, Arango-Lasprilla JC, Vázquez-Barquero A. Epidemiology of Idiopathic Normal Pressure Hydrocephalus: A Systematic Review of the Literature. World Neurosurg. Dec 2015;84(6):2002-9.

13. Hertel F, Walter C, Schmitt M, Mörsdorf M, Jammers W, Busch HP, Bettag M. Is a combination of Tc-SPECT or perfusion weighted magnetic resonance imaging with spinal tap test helpful in the diagnosis of normal pressure hydrocephalus? J Neurol Neurosurg Psychiatry. Apr 2003;74(4):479-84.

14. Woodworth GF, McGirt MJ, Williams MA, Rigamonti D. Cerebrospinal fluid drainage and dynamics in the diagnosis of normal pressure hydrocephalus. Neurosurgery. May 2009;64(5):919-25; discussion 925-926.

15. Algin O, Hakyemez B, Ocakoglu G, Parlak M. MR cisternography: is it useful in the diagnosis of normal-pressure hydrocephalus and the selection of "good shunt responders"? Diagn Interv Radiol Ank Turk. June 2011;17(2):105-11.

16. Campos-Juanatey F, Gutiérrez-Baños JL, Portillo-Martín JA, Zubillaga-Guerrero S. Assessment of the urodynamic diagnosis in patients with urinary incontinence associated with normal pressure hydrocephalus. Neurourol Urodyn. June 2015;34(5):465-8.

17. Czosnyka Z, Owler B, Keong N, Santarius T, Baledent O, Pickard JD, Czosnyka M. Impact of duration of symptoms on CSF dynamics in idiopathic normal pressure hydrocephalus. Acta Neurol Scand. June 2011;123(6):414-8.

18. Vakili S, Moran D, Hung A, Elder BD, Jeon L, Fialho H, Sankey EW, Jusué-Torres I, Goodwin CR, Lu J, Robison J, Rigamonti D. Timing of surgical treatment for idiopathic normal pressure hydrocephalus: association between treatment delay and reduced short-term benefit. Neurosurg Focus. Sep 2016;41(3):E2.

19. Adams RD, Fisher CM, Hakim S, Ojemann RG, Sweet WH. SYMPTOMATIC OCCULT HYDROCEPHALUS WITH "NORMAL" CEREBROSPINAL FLUID PRESSURE.A TREATABLE SYNDROME. N Engl J Med. 15 Jul 1965;273:117-26.

20. Nassar BR, Lippa CF. Idiopathic Normal Pressure Hydrocephalus: A Review for General Practitioners. Gerontol Geriatr Med. 1 Jan 2016;2:2333721416643702.

21. Kubo Y, Kazui H, Yoshida T, Kito Y, Kimura N, Tokunaga H, Ogino A, Miyake H, Ishikawa M, Takeda M. Validation of Grading Scale for Evaluating Symptoms of Idiopathic Normal-Pressure Hydrocephalus. Dement Geriatr Cogn Disord. 20 nov 2007;25(1):37-45.

22. Meier U, Zeilinger FS, Kintzel D. Signs, Symptoms and Course of Normal Pressure Hydrocephalus in Comparison with Cerebral Atrophy. Acta Neurochir (Wien). 1 Oct 1999;141(10):1039-48.

23. Savolainen S, Hurskainen H, Paljärvi L, Alafuzoff I, Vapalahti M. Five-Year Outcome of Normal Pressure Hydrocephalus with or Without a Shunt: Predictive Value of the Clinical Signs, Neuropsychological Evaluation and Infusion Test. Acta Neurochir (Wien). 1 June 2002;144(6):515-23.

24. Krzastek SC, Bruch WM, Robinson SP, Young HF, Klausner AP. Characterization of lower urinary tract symptoms in patients with idiopathic normal pressure hydrocephalus. Neurourol Urodyn. Apr 2017;36(4):1167-73.

25. Fournier JY, Hildebrandt G, Gautschi O. Hydrocephalus at normal pressure. Rev Med Suisse. 21 Apr 2010;245(6):836-9.

26. Bech RA, Waldemar G, Gjerris F, Klinken L, Juhler M. Shunting effects in patients with idiopathic normal pressure hydrocephalus; correlation with cerebral and leptomeningeal biopsy findings. Acta Neurochir (Wien). 1999;141(6):633-9.

27. Kobayashi E, Kanno S, Kawakami N, Narita W, Saito M, Endo K, Iwasaki M, Kawaguchi T, Yamada S, Ishii K, Kazui H, Miyajima M, Ishikawa M, Mori E, Tominaga T, Tanaka F, Suzuki K. Risk factors for unfavourable outcomes after shunt surgery in patients with idiopathic normal-pressure hydrocephalus. Sci Rep. 17 August 2022;12:13921.

28. Pyykkö OT, Nerg O, Niskasaari HM, Niskasaari T, Koivisto AM, Hiltunen M, Pihlajamäki J, Rauramaa T, Kojoukhova M, Alafuzoff I, Soininen H, Jääskeläinen JE, Leinonen V. Incidence, Comorbidities, and Mortality in Idiopathic Normal Pressure Hydrocephalus. World Neurosurg. Apr 2018;112:e624-31.

29. Jacobs L. Diabetes mellitus in normal pressure hydrocephalus. J Neurol Neurosurg Psychiatry. Apr 1977;40(4):331-5.

30. Mirzayan MJ, Luetjens G, Borremans JJ, Regel JP, Krauss JK. Extended long- term (> 5 years) outcome of cerebrospinal fluid shunting in idiopathic normal pressure hydrocephalus. Neurosurgery. August 2010;67(2):295-301.

31. Israelsson H, Carlberg B, Wikkelsö C, Laurell K, Kahlon B, Leijon G, Eklund A, Malm J. Vascular risk factors in INPH. Neurology. 7 Feb 2017;88(6):577-85.

32. Damasceno BP. Neuroimaging in normal pressure hydrocephalus. Dement Neuropsychol. 2015;9(4):350-5.

33. Krauss JK, Regel JP. The predictive value of ventricular CSF removal in normal pressure hydrocephalus. Neurol Res. August 1997;19(4):357-60.

34. Lim TS, Yong SW, Moon SY. Repetitive lumbar punctures as treatment for normal pressure hydrocephalus. Eur Neurol. 2009;62(5):293-7.

35. Williams MA, Malm J. Diagnosis and Treatment of Idiopathic Normal Pressure Hydrocephalus. Contin Lifelong Learn Neurol. Apr 2016;22(2 Dementia):579-99.

36. Alvi MA, Brown D, Yolcu Y, Zreik J, Javeed S, Bydon M, Cutsforth-Gregory JK, Graff-Radford J, Jones DT, Graff-Radford NR, Cogswell PM, Elder BD. Prevalence and Trends in Management of Idiopathic Normal Pressure Hydrocephalus in the United States: Insights from the National Inpatient

Sample. World Neurosurg. 1 Jan 2021;145:e38-52.

37. Komolafe EO, Adeolu AA, Komolafe MA. Treatment of cerebrospinal fluid shunting complications in a Nigerian neurosurgery programme. Case illustrations and review. Pediatr Neurosurg. 2008;44(1):36-42.

38. Toma AK, Papadopoulos MC, Stapleton S, Kitchen ND, Watkins LD. Systematic review of the outcome of shunt surgery in idiopathic normal-pressure hydrocephalus. Acta Neurochir (Wien). oct 2013;155(10):1977-80.

39. Foo NP, Tun YC, Chang CC, Lin HL, Cheng CH, Chuang HY. Clinical Outcome and Safety of Lumboperitoneal Shunt in the Treatment of Non-Obstructive Hydrocephalus. Clin Interv Aging. 23 March 2023;18:477-83.

40. Yin R, Zhang X, Wei JJ, Chang JB, Chen YH, Xu HS, Li PT, Yang L, Liu XY, Wang RZ. [Efficacy and outcomes of shunt surgery for secondary hydrocephalus]. Zhonghua Yi Xue Za Zhi. 4 Jul 2023;103(25):1936-9.

41. Klinge P, Marmarou A, Bergsneider M, Relkin N, Black PM. Outcome of shunting in idiopathic normal-pressure hydrocephalus and the value of outcome assessment in shunted patients. Neurosurgery. Sept 2005;57(3 Suppl):S40-52; discussion ii-v.

42. Tisell M, Hellström P, Ahl-Börjesson G, Barrows G, Blomsterwall E, Tullberg M, Wikkelsö C. Long-term outcome in 109 adult patients operated on for hydrocephalus. Br J Neurosurg. August 2006;20(4):214-21.

43. Hebb AO, Cusimano MD. Idiopathic normal pressure hydrocephalus: a systematic review of diagnosis and outcome. Neurosurgery. Nov 2001;49(5):1166-84; discussion 1184-1186.

44. Zaccaria V, Bacigalupo I, Gervasi G, Canevelli M, Corbo M, Vanacore N, Lacorte E. A systematic review on the epidemiology of normal pressure hydrocephalus. Acta Neurol Scand. Feb 2020;141(2):101-14.

45. Táborský J, Blažková J, Beneš V. The Epidemiology of Normal Pressure Hydrocephalus. In: Bradac O, editor. Normal Pressure Hydrocephalus: Pathophysiology, Diagnosis, Treatment and Outcome [Internet]. Cham: Springer International Publishing; 2023 [cited 26 Feb 2024]. p. 39-51. Available from: https://doi.org/10.1007/978-3-031-36522-5_4

46. Oertel JMK, Huelser MJM. Predicting the outcome of normal pressure hydrocephalus therapy-where do we stand? Acta Neurochir (Wien). 1 March 2021;163(3):767-9.

47. Kimura T, Yamada S, Sugimura T, Seki T, Miyano M, Fukuda S, Takeuchi S, Miyata S, Tucker A, Fujita T, Hashizume A, Izumi N, Kawasaki K, Nakagaki A, Sako K. Preoperative Predictive Factors of Short-Term Outcome in Idiopathic Normal Pressure Hydrocephalus. World Neurosurg. Jul 2021;151:e399-406.

48. Marmarou A, Young HF, Aygok GA, Sawauchi S, Tsuji O, Yamamoto T, Dunbar
J. Diagnosis and management of idiopathic normal-pressure hydrocephalus: a prospective study in 151 patients. J Neurosurg. June 2005;102(6):987-97.

49. Walchenbach R, Geiger E, Thomeer RTWM, Vanneste J a. L. The value of temporary external lumbar CSF drainage in predicting the outcome of shunting on normal pressure hydrocephalus. J Neurol Neurosurg Psychiatry. Apr 2002;72(4):503-6.

50. Agostini V, Lanotte M, Carlone M, Campagnoli M, Azzolin I, Scarafia R, Massazza G, Knaflitz M. Instrumented gait analysis for an objective pre/postassessment of tap test in normal pressure hydrocephalus. Arch Phys Med Rehabil. Jul 2015;96(7):1235-41.

51. Marmarou A, Bergsneider M, Klinge P, Relkin N, Black PM. The value of supplemental prognostic tests for the preoperative assessment of idiopathic

normal-pressure hydrocephalus. Neurosurgery. Sept 2005;57(3 Suppl):S17-28; discussion ii-v.

52. Mongin M, Hommet C, Mondon K. Hydrocephalus at normal pressure: update and practical aspects. Rev Médecine Interne. 1 Dec 2015;36(12):825-33.

53. Ishikawa M, Hashimoto M, Mori E, Kuwana N, Kazui H. The value of the cerebrospinal fluid tap test for predicting shunt effectiveness in idiopathic normal pressure hydrocephalus. Fluids Barriers CNS. 13 Jan 2012;9:1.

54. da Rocha SFB, Kowacs PA, de Souza RKM, Pedro MKF, Ramina R, Teive HAG. Serial Tap Test of patients with idiopathic normal pressure hydrocephalus: impact on cognitive function and its meaning. Fluids Barriers CNS. May 6, 2021;18:22.

55. Andrén K, Wikkelsö C, Sundström N, Agerskov S, Israelsson H, Laurell K, Hellström P, Tullberg M. Long-term effects of complications and vascular comorbidity in idiopathic normal pressure hydrocephalus: a quality registry study. J Neurol. 2018;265(1):178-86.

56. Klinge P, Hellström P, Tans J, Wikkelsø C, European iNPH Multicentre Study Group. One-year outcome in the European multicentre study on iNPH. Acta Neurol Scand. Sept 2012;126(3):145-53.

57. Folstein MF, Folstein SE, McHugh PR. "Mini-mental state. A practical method for grading the cognitive state of patients for the clinician. J Psychiatr Res. Nov 1975;12(3):189-98.

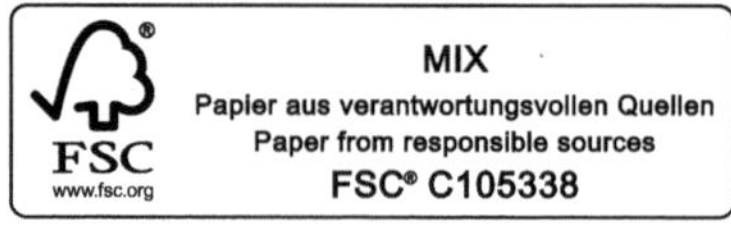

Printed by Books on Demand GmbH, Norderstedt / Germany